Sardine Diet

A Beginner's Quick Start Guide on Its Health Benefits, With Sample Curated Recipes and a Meal Plan

mf

copyright © 2023 Bruce Ackerberg

All rights reserved No part of this book may be reproduced, or stored in a retrieval system, or transmitted in any form or by any means, electronic, mechanical, photocopying, recording, or otherwise, without express written permission of the publisher.

Disclaimer

By reading this disclaimer, you are accepting the terms of the disclaimer in full. If you disagree with this disclaimer, please do not read the guide.

All of the content within this guide is provided for informational and educational purposes only, and should not be accepted as independent medical or other professional advice. The author is not a doctor, physician, nurse, mental health provider, or registered nutritionist/dietician. Therefore, using and reading this guide does not establish any form of a physician-patient relationship.

Always consult with a physician or another qualified health provider with any issues or questions you might have regarding any sort of medical condition. Do not ever disregard any qualified professional medical advice or delay seeking that advice because of anything you have read in this guide. The information in this guide is not intended to be any sort of medical advice and should not be used in lieu of any medical advice by a licensed and qualified medical professional.

The information in this guide has been compiled from a variety of known sources. However, the author cannot attest to or guarantee the accuracy of each source and thus should not be held liable for any errors or omissions.

You acknowledge that the publisher of this guide will not be held liable for any loss or damage of any kind incurred as a result of this guide or the reliance on any information provided within this guide. You acknowledge and agree that you assume all risk and responsibility for any action you undertake in response to the information in this guide.

Using this guide does not guarantee any particular result (e.g., weight loss or a cure). By reading this guide, you acknowledge that there are no guarantees to any specific outcome or results you can expect.

All product names, diet plans, or names used in this guide are for identification purposes only and are the property of their respective owners. The use of these names does not imply endorsement. All other trademarks cited herein are the property of their respective owners.

Where applicable, this guide is not intended to be a substitute for the original work of this diet plan and is, at most, a supplement to the original work of this diet plan and never a direct substitute. This guide is a personal expression of the facts of that diet plan.

Where applicable, persons shown in the cover images are stock photography models and the publisher has obtained the rights to use the images through license agreements with third-party stock image companies.

Table of Contents

Introduction 7
What Is a Sardine Diet? 9
    Common Concerns and Myths About Sardines 9
    Benefits of the Sardine 12
    Disadvantages of the Sardine Diet 17
Grocery Tips for Buying Sardines 20
    Freshness is key 20
    Check the packaging 21
    Read the labels 21
    Consider the source 22
    Opt for fresh or frozen 23
    Reputable brands known in sardines 24
Step-Guide on How to Get Started with Sardine Diet 27
    Step 1: Choose your sardines 27
    Step 2: Incorporate sardines into meals 28
    Step 3: Balance your diet 29
    Incorporating Sardines into Your Meals 30
    Why Adding Sardines Can Be Easy? 33
Sample Recipes 36
    Sardine Toast with Tomato and Sweet Onion 37
    Sardine and Avocado Salad 38
    Sardine Pasta with Garlic and Lemon 39
    Sardine and White Bean Dip 40
    Sardine and Cucumber Salad 41
    Sardine and Olive Tapenade 42
    Grilled Sardines with Herbs 43
    Sardine and Tomato Bruschetta 44
    Sardine and Spinach Stuffed Portobello Mushrooms .. 45
    Sardine and Potato Croquettes 46

Sardine and Tomato Pizza	47
Sardine Tacos with Mango Salsa	48
Sardine and Rice Stuffed Bell Peppers	49
Sardine and Roasted Pepper Sandwich	50
Sardine and Lemon Risotto	51
7-Day Meal Plan	**52**
Day 1	52
Day 2	52
Day 3	52
Day 4	53
Day 5	53
Day 6	53
Day 7	53
Conclusion	**55**
FAQs	**58**
Resources and Helpful Links	**62**

Introduction

There are a lot of healthy options to choose from for anyone who wants to try out different ways to lose weight or improve their food options for their health. One of which is choosing to focus on a pescatarian diet. One of which is following a sardine diet.

Sardines may be small, but they pack a powerful nutritional punch. Rich in omega-3 fatty acids, protein, vitamins, and minerals, sardines offer a wealth of benefits for both your body and mind. Incorporating sardines into your diet can improve heart health, boost brain function, aid in weight management, and promote overall well-being.

Imagine feeling more energetic, sharper mentally, and having a strengthened immune system. With the sardine diet, you can achieve all of this and more. Not only will you be nourishing your body with essential nutrients, but you will also be savoring every bite with the delicious taste of fresh sardines.

In this guide, we will talk about the following;

- What is a Sardine Diet?

- Common concerns and myths about sardines
- Benefits of the Sardine Diet
- Disadvantages of the Sardine Diet
- How to get started with the Sardine Diet
- Grocery shopping tips on how to buy sardines
- Reputable brands known in sardines
- Sample recipes and sample meal plan

With this guide, you will be able to get started on your sardine journey today. Not only will you be given different ways to select and prepare sardines in your meals, this guide will also help you navigate how to start, follow, and keep a healthy sardine diet.

What Is a Sardine Diet?

A sardine diet is a meal plan that emphasizes the inclusion of sardines in your meals. This type of diet is gaining popularity due to its myriad of health benefits and the delectable taste it offers. Sardines, being small and oily fish, are not only rich in essential nutrients like omega-3 fatty acids, protein, vitamins, and minerals, but they also provide a significant source of calcium and phosphorus, promoting bone health and strength.

Additionally, the omega-3 fatty acids found in sardines have been linked to reducing inflammation, improving heart health, and supporting brain function. With their versatility and nutritional value, sardines are an excellent choice for those looking to enhance their overall well-being through a delicious and wholesome dietary approach.

Common Concerns and Myths About Sardines

Despite all the health benefits of sardines, there are still some common concerns or myths about them. Many people worry that consuming sardines will result in mercury poisoning due to their environment and high levels of omega-3 fatty acids.

However, this is not true as long as you buy high-quality sardines from reputable brands and consume them in moderation. Here are some myths and facts about sardines;

1. *Concern:* Sardines have a strong fishy taste and smell.
   Fact: While sardines do have a distinct flavor, their taste is often milder compared to other fish varieties. This mildness allows for a versatile culinary experience, as the rich, savory notes of sardines are appreciated by many seafood enthusiasts. Whether grilled to perfection, marinated in zesty sauces, or added to a hearty pasta dish, sardines offer a delightful addition to any meal. If you're new to sardines, don't hesitate to experiment with different cooking methods and recipes to find a preparation style that perfectly suits your palate.

2. *Concern:* Sardines are high in mercury and should be avoided.
   Fact: Sardines, known as low-mercury fish, are a safe choice for regular consumption due to their lower position on the food chain. Unlike larger predatory fish like tuna or swordfish, sardines accumulate fewer toxins, including mercury. As a result, they provide an excellent source of omega-3 fatty acids without the associated concerns of mercury contamination.

Incorporating sardines into your diet can offer a nutritious and sustainable option for enhancing your omega-3 intake.

3. *Concern:* Eating sardines can cause bones to get stuck in the throat.
   Fact: Sardines, those delicious little fish, are typically sold in convenient canned form. One unique feature of sardines is that their bones are usually soft and edible, which adds to their nutritional value. These tiny fish are not only packed with protein, but they also provide the added benefit of being rich in calcium and other essential minerals. However, if you prefer boneless sardines, worry not! You can easily find boneless options in many stores, ensuring a hassle-free culinary experience. So go ahead and indulge in the goodness of sardines, knowing that you have both options available to suit your preferences!

4. *Concern:* Sardines are not sustainable and contribute to overfishing.
   Fact: When it comes to selecting sardines, it is crucial to opt for sustainably sourced options that contribute to the well-being of fish populations. To ensure you make an environmentally responsible choice, look for reputable brands that adhere to sustainable fishing practices and possess certifications such as the Marine Stewardship Council (MSC) label. By supporting

sustainable fishing, we are actively safeguarding the long-term viability of sardine populations and promoting the health of marine ecosystems for generations to come.

5. _Myth:_ Sardines are unhealthy due to their oil content.
   Fact: Sardines, those small and flavorful fish, are not only delicious but also packed with numerous health benefits. The oil found in sardines is rich in omega-3 fatty acids, including EPA and DHA, which are well-known for their positive impact on heart health, brain function, and reducing inflammation throughout the body. These healthy fats not only help maintain good cholesterol levels but also promote optimal cognitive function and support overall well-being. By including sardines in your balanced diet, you can easily incorporate this powerhouse of nutrients into your meals and reap the rewards of their remarkable nutritional profile.

By debunking these common concerns and myths, we can appreciate sardines for their unique flavor, nutritional benefits, and sustainability. Including sardines in your diet can be a delicious and healthy choice.

Benefits of the Sardine

The health benefits of the sardine diet are numerous, ranging from improved heart health to enhanced mental sharpness.

Here is a closer look at some of the remarkable advantages you can experience when incorporating sardines into your meals:

Rich in Omega-3 Fatty Acids

Sardines are an excellent source of omega-3 fatty acids, making them a valuable addition to any diet. These essential fats are known for their ability to support heart health by reducing levels of triglycerides and LDL cholesterol. Additionally, omega-3 fatty acids have anti-inflammatory properties that can help reduce joint pain and inflammation throughout the body.

Brain Health

Following that, omega-3 fatty acids have been proven to boost cognitive function, memory, and overall brain health and function. Research studies have shown that omega-3s may help reduce the risk of cognitive decline and dementia at one age. Omega-3 deficiency is a common cause of mental health issues such as depression, anxiety, and mood disorders.

Some studies also suggest that omega-3s could help protect against age-related macular degeneration, a leading cause of blindness. Consuming sardines as a part of a healthy diet may help promote brain health and improve the overall quality of life, especially in older adults.

High in Protein

Sardines are also an excellent source of high-quality protein. Protein is necessary for many body processes, including the development and repair of tissues, the support of muscular growth, and the preservation of general health.

It plays a crucial role in the formation of enzymes, hormones, and antibodies. By including sardines in your diet, you can ensure an adequate intake of protein, promoting tissue repair, muscle development, and optimal functioning of your body's systems.

Abundant in Vitamins and Minerals

Sardines contain essential nutrients like vitamin B12, which plays a vital role in nerve function and the production of red blood cells. Minerals such as calcium and phosphorus, which are crucial for maintaining strong and healthy bones, are also present.

Additionally, they provide selenium, an important mineral that supports energy metabolism and immune function. By including sardines in your diet, you can ensure a diverse intake of these essential vitamins and minerals, contributing to overall health and well-being.

Good for Weight Management

Sardines are an excellent option for those looking to manage their weight as they offer a range of benefits. A single serving of canned sardines contains roughly 25 grams of protein while providing approximately 150 calories. This high protein content helps promote feelings of fullness and satisfaction, thereby preventing unnecessary snacking or overeating.

Just as mentioned above, sardines are also a good source of omega-3 fatty acids, which are crucial for maintaining a healthy weight. These fatty acids can stimulate fat-burning enzymes, leading to a more efficient metabolism. Along with this, sardines are a low-fat, low-calorie food that provides an excellent source of various vitamins and minerals, including vitamin D, calcium, and phosphorus.

Supportive Heart Health

Incorporating sardines into one's diet can provide numerous benefits for heart health. The omega-3 fatty acids found in these small fish have been shown to have cholesterol-lowering effects, which can ultimately reduce the risk of heart disease.

Studies have indicated that consuming sardines can improve overall cardiovascular health by regulating blood pressure and reducing inflammation. Sardines are also a great source of protein, which can contribute to maintaining a healthy weight and reducing the risk of obesity, another risk factor for heart disease.

Bone Health

Sardines are a powerhouse of essential nutrients that contribute to maintaining optimal bone health. They are an excellent source of calcium, a mineral that forms the basic foundation of bones, along with other minerals such as phosphorus and magnesium. In addition, sardines are abundant in vitamin D, which facilitates calcium absorption and regulates the body's balance of calcium and phosphorus.

Studies have also shown that omega-3 fatty acids present in sardines can reduce the risk of bone loss and improve bone density. Incorporating sardines into one's diet is an easy and delicious way to benefit from their bone-strengthening properties.

Anti-Inflammatory Properties

The anti-inflammatory properties of sardines are well documented and greatly benefit those suffering from chronic diseases such as arthritis and asthma. The omega-3 fatty acids found in sardines have been shown to reduce inflammation in the body, limiting the occurrence of inflammation-related illnesses. Furthermore, the antioxidants in sardines help to neutralize free radicals that contribute to oxidative stress that is known to trigger the body's inflammatory response.

This makes sardines an excellent dietary source of anti-inflammatory properties to help manage chronic inflammation diseases. Additionally, their high protein content, low mercury levels, and cost-effectiveness make sardines an attractive addition to an anti-inflammatory diet.

Incorporating sardines into your diet can provide a wide array of health benefits, making them a valuable addition to a balanced and nutritious eating plan.

Disadvantages of the Sardine Diet

While the benefits of a sardine diet generally outweigh the disadvantages, it's important to consider potential drawbacks. Here are some disadvantages associated with a sardine diet:

Strong Odor

This is a common complaint among people who want to incorporate them into their diet. This distinct odor is caused by the high levels of trimethylamine oxide present in their flesh, which breaks down into trimethylamine, giving off a pungent smell similar to ammonia.

It's recommended to try rinsing the sardines in cold water before consuming them or pair them with strong flavors like lemon, garlic, or chili peppers to mask the smell.

Mercury Content

Sardines can contain small amounts of mercury that may pose health risks when consumed in excess. Mercury is a toxic metal that can accumulate in fish's flesh and harm the nervous system, leading to cognitive and developmental issues in fetuses, infants, and young children. Pregnant women, nursing mothers, and parents who feed their children sardines should be mindful of the potential risks and limit their intake to no more than two to three servings per week.

Additionally, they can choose canned sardines with lower mercury levels and avoid eating sardines with other high-mercury fish or shellfish. While sardines are undoubtedly a nutritious food option, it's crucial to balance their benefits with their potential drawbacks to promote optimal health and safety.

Allergies and Sensitivities

Individuals with fish allergies or specific sensitivities to proteins found in sardines should be wary of including this fish in their diet. Sardines are rich in omega-3 fatty acids, protein, and other important nutrients. However, some people may experience adverse reactions to sardines, such as itchiness, swelling, and digestive problems.

In severe cases, an allergic reaction can lead to anaphylaxis, a life-threatening condition. Therefore, it's crucial to consult a healthcare professional before trying sardines if you have a known allergy or sensitivity. They can help you determine whether it's safe to incorporate sardines into your diet or suggest alternative sources of nutrition.

Availability and Accessibility

While sardines are widely accessible and can be found in most supermarkets and fishmongers, some parts of the world may not have access to this type of fish due to limited distribution channels and demand. However, even for those who do have access to sardines, a major disadvantage of the sardine diet is its high sodium content. This is especially true for canned sardines, which are often packed in oil or saltwater. Consuming too much sodium can lead to high blood pressure, heart disease, and other health problems.

Individuals who consume sardines regularly need to be mindful of their sodium intake and choose low-sodium options whenever possible. Another consideration is that some people may not enjoy the taste or texture of sardines, which can make it difficult to incorporate them into their diet regularly.

Despite these potential disadvantages, the overall benefits of a sardine diet tend to outweigh the drawbacks. As with any dietary changes, it's recommended to consider individual needs, and preferences, and consult with a healthcare professional or registered dietitian to ensure the diet aligns with your specific circumstances.

Grocery Tips for Buying Sardines

When it comes to selecting high-quality sardines, there are a few factors to consider to ensure freshness and maximize nutritional benefits. Here are some guidance tips:

Freshness is key

When it comes to selecting sardines, freshness should be the top priority. To ensure maximum freshness, it's important to look for sardines that have been recently caught and processed. Fresh sardines are characterized by bright, clear eyes, shiny silver skin, and a firm texture. If you notice an off smell, dull or discolored skin, or cloudy eyes, it's best to avoid buying those sardines altogether.

These signs indicate that the sardines may be less fresh, which could ultimately affect both the taste and nutritional value. It's also useful to note that sardines are rich in omega-3 fatty acids, which provide numerous health benefits, including cognitive function, heart health, and inflammation reduction. Therefore, choosing fresh sardines is not only important for taste but also for maximizing nutritional value.

Check the packaging

When choosing sardines, it is crucial to consider the type of packaging they come in. It is advisable to opt for sardines that are packed in either oil or water because these methods preserve the flavor and texture of the fish. In contrast, sardines packed in heavy sauces or with added preservatives may not only detract from their natural taste but also reduce their nutritional value.

Sardines in oil or water are also typically less salty than those packed in heavy sauces, making them a healthier option. By making a conscious effort to select sardines packed in oil or water, one can ensure that they enjoy the best possible taste while maximizing their nutritional intake.

Read the labels

When selecting sardines, taking a moment to read the label is crucial. It is essential to look for sardines that are sustainably sourced and indicate that they were caught using fishing methods that reduce harm to the environment. Sustainable fishing practices play a significant role in protecting marine ecosystems and ensuring that fish populations are preserved for future generations.

Certifications such as MSC (Marine Stewardship Council) and Friend of the Sea are excellent ways to assure sustainable fishing practices. MSC is a globally recognized certification program that assesses fisheries and ensures they are meeting specific sustainability standards. Friend of the Sea verifies that seafood products come from sustainable fisheries that adhere to rigorous sustainability criteria.

It is important to note that unsustainable fishing practices have contributed to the decline of many fish populations worldwide. Therefore, selecting sustainably sourced sardines can be a small but essential step to promote responsible consumption and preserve the environment.

Consider the source

To ensure the best flavor and nutritional profile, it is recommended to choose sardines sourced from cold, clean waters. Cold waters promote the accumulation of healthy omega-3 fatty acids in sardines, making them an excellent source of vital nutrients for maintaining a healthy diet. Additionally, sardines sourced from clean waters have reduced exposure to environmental toxins that may accumulate in their flesh.

To ensure that you are consuming the highest quality sardines, look for reputable brands known for their commitment to quality and sustainable fishing practices. These brands are typically transparent about their sourcing and production methods, ensuring that you feel confident when choosing a product. By selecting sardines from reputable brands and sources, you can enjoy a delicious, healthy snack with peace of mind.

Opt for fresh or frozen

Fresh or frozen sardines are the best options to choose from because of their exceptional flavor and nutritional value. Fresh sardines can be found at fish markets or specialty seafood stores and are highly recommended for those who desire a more intense and delightful taste. These fish are rich in omega-3 fatty acids, minerals such as potassium, magnesium, and iron, and vitamins B12 and D.

On the other hand, frozen sardines are a practical option. They can also retain their nutritional value and taste when thawed properly. Proper thawing is crucial to avoid losing the natural oils, which contribute to the flavor and nutritional content of the fish. Therefore, always follow the manufacturer's guidelines for thawing to ensure the fish's quality is maintained. Whether fresh or frozen, sardines are an excellent choice for those seeking a nutrient-rich, delicious, and easy-to-prepare meal.

Remember, sardines are delicate fish, so proper storage is crucial to maintain their freshness. Once opened, store any leftover sardines in an airtight container in the refrigerator and consume them within a day or two for optimal taste and quality.

By following these tips, you can select high-quality sardines that not only taste delicious but also provide the maximum nutritional benefits for your sardine diet.

Reputable brands known in sardines

When it comes to reputable brands known for their quality sardine products, here are a few options:

Wild Planet

Wild Planet is a reputable brand that offers sustainably sourced sardines that are packed in either extra virgin olive oil or water. They prioritize ethical and environmentally responsible fishing practices, ensuring high-quality products for their consumers. Their sardines are caught using pole and troll methods, minimizing the impact on non-targeted species.

Additionally, their packaging is BPA-free and recyclable. Wild Planet's commitment to sustainable fishing practices and eco-friendly packaging demonstrates its dedication to both the health of the consumer and the environment.

King Oscar

King Oscar is a reputable brand in the world of canned seafood, specifically sardines. With over 100 years of experience in the industry, they have solidified their position as one of the most trusted and highest-quality producers of sardines.

Their products come in a variety of flavors and are packed with premium ingredients such as olive oil or tomato sauce. King Oscar's commitment to flavor and quality has made them a go-to choice for seafood lovers around the globe.

Matiz

Matiz is a reputable Spanish brand that offers a wide array of high-quality seafood products, with sardines being their specialty. Sourced from the Galician coast of Spain, Matiz's sardines are known for their authenticity and exquisite taste. These sardines are hand-packed in premium olive oil, giving them a delightful and distinct flavor. The brand prides itself on its commitment to sourcing sustainably caught sardines while maintaining fair trade practices.

Furthermore, Matiz's sardines are packed in a variety of formats, including tins, jars, and pouches, making them convenient for customers to enjoy anytime, anywhere. With a focus on both quality and sustainability, Matiz has earned its reputation as a top-notch brand for sardines.

Bela

Bela is a reputable brand known for producing high-quality sardines that are sustainably caught and packed in organic extra virgin olive oil. Bela sardines are a delicious and nutritious option for sardine enthusiasts as they are rich in protein, omega-3 fatty acids, and essential vitamins and minerals.

The brand takes pride in its sustainable fishing practices, ensuring that its sardines are caught responsibly to minimize the impact on the marine ecosystem. Bela also ensures that their olive oil is of the highest quality, providing a flavorful and healthy complement to their sardines. With their commitment to sustainability and quality, Bela is a top choice for those looking for a premium sardine experience.

Remember, availability may vary depending on your location, so it's a good idea to check local specialty stores or online retailers for these brands. Additionally, reading customer reviews can help you gauge the overall satisfaction and quality of the products.

Keep in mind that while these brands are reputable, personal preferences may vary. It's always a good idea to try different brands to find the one that suits your taste and dietary preferences best.

Step-Guide on How to Get Started with Sardine Diet

Getting started with the sardine diet doesn't have to be difficult. Here are a few tips and tricks to help you make the transition simple and enjoyable:

Step 1: Choose your sardines

When you choose sardines for your diet, it's important to opt for sustainably sourced options, whether they are canned or fresh. Look for sardines that are packed in water or olive oil instead of heavy sauces to minimize the number of added ingredients. By selecting sustainably sourced sardines, you're supporting responsible fishing practices and helping to preserve marine ecosystems.

Sardines packed in water or olive oil offer a more natural and healthier option compared to those packed in heavy sauces. This allows you to fully appreciate the flavors and nutritional benefits of the sardines without unnecessary additives. Plus, water or olive oil-packed sardines tend to have a cleaner taste, making them versatile for various recipes.

When shopping for sardines, check the labels and packaging for information on sustainability certifications or eco-friendly practices. Look for brands that prioritize sustainable fishing methods and ensure the long-term health of fish populations.

By consciously choosing sustainably sourced sardines and those packed in water or olive oil, you can enjoy the many benefits of this nutritious fish while also contributing to a more sustainable food system.

Step 2: Incorporate sardines into meals

When it comes to incorporating sardines into your meals, the options are plentiful! You can try enjoying them straight out of the can for a quick and convenient snack that's packed with nutrition. The natural flavors of sardines make them delicious on their own.

For a boost of protein and flavor, consider adding sardines to salads. Whether it's a refreshing green salad or a hearty grain salad, sardines can provide a satisfying and nutritious addition. Their rich and savory taste pairs well with various salad ingredients, such as leafy greens, tomatoes, cucumbers, and olives.

If you're feeling adventurous in the kitchen, get creative with sardine recipes. Use them to make flavorful fish cakes or fritters. Combine mashed sardines with breadcrumbs, herbs, and spices, then pan-fry until golden and crispy. These make for a tasty appetizer or main dish.

Don't be afraid to experiment with different flavors and culinary techniques to find your preferred way of enjoying sardines. Consider incorporating them into pasta dishes, sandwiches, or even as a topping for pizzas. The possibilities are endless!

By exploring different ways to incorporate sardines into your meals, you can discover new and exciting flavors while reaping the nutritional benefits they offer. Remember to have fun in the kitchen and let your taste buds guide you on this delicious journey.

Step 3: Balance your diet

When it comes to maintaining a healthy diet, incorporating sardines is just one piece of the puzzle. To ensure you're meeting all your nutritional needs, it's important to maintain a balanced and varied diet overall.

Include a wide variety of fruits and vegetables in your meals. These colorful powerhouses are rich in essential vitamins, minerals, and antioxidants, which contribute to overall health and well-being. Opt for a rainbow of produce to ensure you're getting a range of nutrients.

Whole grains should also be a part of your balanced diet. They provide fiber, B vitamins, and minerals. Incorporate whole wheat bread, brown rice, quinoa, or oats into your meals to add variety and promote good digestion.

Lean proteins such as poultry, fish, tofu, and legumes are vital for building and repairing tissues, as well as supporting a healthy immune system. Sardines offer an excellent source of omega-3 fatty acids and protein, but it's important to diversify your protein sources to meet all your nutritional requirements.

To maintain balance, limit processed foods, sugary snacks, and unhealthy fats. Instead, focus on nutrient-dense options that nourish your body. Drink plenty of water to stay hydrated and support optimal bodily functions.

By including a variety of fruits, vegetables, whole grains, lean proteins, and sardines in your meals, you'll ensure that you're providing your body with the necessary nutrients it needs to thrive. Remember, balance is key to achieving optimal health and wellness.

Incorporating sardines into your diet can be beneficial for your health and provide a flavorful way to support sustainable fishing practices. With these tips and tricks, you'll be well on your way to enjoying all the benefits of a sardine-enriched diet!

Incorporating Sardines into Your Meals

Sardines can be enjoyed in various ways, whether you have fresh or canned options at hand. Their versatility makes them a great addition to a wide range of recipes. Here are some ideas on how to incorporate sardines into your meals:

1. **Salads:** Sardines are a great addition to any salad, providing a boost of protein and a punch of flavor. For a delicious and healthy meal, simply add them to your favorite greens, along with some juicy tomatoes and crunchy cucumbers, then finish with a drizzle of fresh lemon juice or vinaigrette dressing.

2. **Wraps and sandwiches:** Create mouthwatering wraps or sandwiches bursting with flavor by combining succulent sardines with an array of fresh vegetables, such as crisp lettuce, creamy avocado, and juicy sliced tomatoes. For an extra layer of delectable taste, indulge in a spread like zesty pesto or creamy mayo. Elevate your culinary experience with these delightful combinations that will leave your taste buds craving for more.

3. **Rice bowls:** Sardines, with their rich flavor and delicate texture, can be a delectable addition to rice bowls. Picture this: a bed of fluffy, perfectly cooked rice topped with succulent sardines, accompanied by an array of vibrant steamed vegetables bursting with color and nutrients. To elevate the dish even further, drizzle your favorite sauce or sprinkle a touch of your preferred seasoning to create a symphony of flavors. This quick and nutritious meal will surely satisfy your

taste buds and leave you feeling nourished and satisfied.

4. **Pasta dishes:** To add a Mediterranean twist to your pasta dishes, consider incorporating sardines. These small, flavorful fish can elevate your meal with their unique taste and texture. Simply combine them with al dente pasta, drizzle with extra virgin olive oil, sautéed garlic, and a sprinkle of lemon zest for a burst of freshness. To enhance the flavors even further, you can also add aromatic herbs like parsley or basil. This combination of ingredients creates a delicious and satisfying dish that is sure to impress your taste buds.

5. **Sardine toasts:** Start your day with a delightful breakfast option by toasting a slice of bread to perfection. Then, generously spread a scrumptious mixture of mashed sardines, zesty lemon juice, fragrant fresh herbs, and a sprinkle of sea salt on top. This simple yet delicious combination offers a burst of flavors that can be enjoyed not only for breakfast but also for a satisfying lunch or a light snack throughout the day. Treat your taste buds to this delectable and versatile dish!

The ease of incorporating sardines into your existing meal plans is one of their advantages. Whether you choose fresh sardines or opt for the convenience of canned ones, they can add nutritional value and flavor to your dishes. Don't be afraid to experiment and explore different recipes to find your favorite way to enjoy sardines.

Why Adding Sardines Can Be Easy?

Incorporating sardines into your existing meal plans is incredibly easy due to their versatility and convenience. Here are a few reasons why adding sardines to your diet can be a seamless process:

Quick and Convenient

Sardines offer a quick and easy way to add healthy protein and Omega-3 fatty acids to your diet. They require no preparation time and can be eaten straight from the tin, making them perfect for busy individuals. Sardines can even be incorporated into various meals, including salads, sandwiches, and pasta dishes, for added flavor and nutrition.

Furthermore, they are inexpensive and have a longer shelf life than fresh fish. With so many benefits, it's no wonder that adding sardines to your diet can be a seamless process.

Minimal Cooking Required

Sardines are an ideal addition to meals when time is limited. With fresher sardines, cooking is quick and effortless, taking just a few minutes of grilling, broiling, or pan-frying. They contain no scales or bones, making them a simple ingredient that requires minimal preparation. Sardines are also packed with nutrients and omega-3 fatty acids, making them not only a fast and easy option but a healthy one as well.

Versatile Flavor Profile

Sardines, with their rich and distinctive flavor, offer a delightful culinary experience that adds depth and character to a variety of dishes. Whether tossed in a vibrant salad, nestled between layers of a hearty sandwich, mixed with al dente pasta, or wrapped in a flavorful tortilla, these little fish provide a burst of flavor that elevates every bite.

Their unique taste, combined with their versatility, makes them a perfect complement to a wide range of ingredients and cuisines, allowing for endless creative possibilities in the kitchen.

Nutrient Boost

Sardines are a nutritional powerhouse, offering an impressive array of nutrients. They are packed with high-quality protein, essential vitamins, and minerals. Notably, sardines are an excellent source of omega-3 fatty acids, known for their role in supporting brain health and reducing inflammation in the body.

Furthermore, their rich Vitamin D content aids in calcium absorption, contributing to stronger bones and teeth. Including sardines in your diet can provide a wide range of health benefits to support overall well-being.

Suitable for Different Diets

Sardines are suitable for a variety of dietary preferences, making them an accessible ingredient regardless of your chosen eating style. Whether you follow a vegan, vegetarian, keto, Paleo, or gluten-free diet, sardines can be an excellent addition to any meal plan.

To incorporate sardines into your meal plans, you can start by replacing other protein sources, such as chicken or beef, with sardines in your favorite recipes. You can also experiment by adding them to salads, wraps, or pasta dishes for a flavorful twist.

Remember to check labels and choose sustainably sourced sardines whenever possible. This ensures that you're making an environmentally responsible choice while enjoying the health benefits of this versatile fish.

Sample Recipes

Sardine Toast with Tomato and Sweet Onion

Ingredients:

- Sardines (canned)
- Tomato
- Sweet onion
- Bread slices

Instructions:

1. Toast the bread slices.
2. Spread the sardines on the toast.
3. Top with sliced tomato and sweet onion.
4. Serve as an appetizer or light meal.

Sardine and Avocado Salad

Ingredients:

- Sardines (canned)
- Avocado
- Lettuce
- Lemon juice
- Olive oil

Instructions:

1. Arrange lettuce leaves on a plate.

2. Top with sardines and avocado slices.

3. Drizzle with lemon juice and olive oil.

4. Season with salt and pepper to taste.

Sardine Pasta with Garlic and Lemon

Ingredients:

- Sardines (canned)
- Pasta
- Garlic cloves
- Lemon
- Olive oil

Instructions:

1. Cook pasta according to package instructions.
2. In a pan, sauté minced garlic in olive oil until fragrant.
3. Add sardines and break them up with a fork.
4. Toss cooked pasta with the sardine mixture.
5. Squeeze fresh lemon juice over the pasta before serving.

Sardine and White Bean Dip

Ingredients:

- Sardines (canned)
- Cannellini beans
- Lemon juice
- Garlic clove
- Olive oil

Instructions:

1. Combine sardines, cannellini beans, lemon juice, and minced garlic in a food processor.

2. Blend until smooth, adding olive oil gradually to achieve desired consistency.

3. Serve as a dip with crackers or vegetable sticks.

Sardine and Cucumber Salad

Ingredients:

- Sardines (canned)
- Cucumber
- Red onion
- Fresh dill
- Greek yogurt

Instructions:

1. Chop cucumber and red onion into small pieces.
2. In a bowl, mix sardines, chopped vegetables, fresh dill, and Greek yogurt.
3. Season with salt and pepper to taste.
4. Serve as a refreshing salad or filling for sandwiches.

Sardine and Olive Tapenade

Ingredients:

- Sardines (canned)
- Black olives
- Capers
- Garlic clove
- Lemon juice

Instructions:

1. In a food processor, combine sardines, black olives, capers, minced garlic, and lemon juice.

2. Pulse until well combined but still slightly chunky.

3. Spread the tapenade on bread or use it as a topping for grilled vegetables.

Grilled Sardines with Herbs

Ingredients:

- Fresh sardines
- Fresh herbs (such as parsley, thyme, or rosemary)
- Lemon wedges
- Olive oil

Instructions:

1. Preheat the grill to medium-high heat.
2. Rub fresh sardines with olive oil and season with salt and pepper.
3. Place sardines on the grill and cook for 3-4 minutes per side.
4. Sprinkle with fresh herbs and serve with lemon wedges.

Sardine and Tomato Bruschetta

Ingredients:

- Sardines (canned)
- Cherry tomatoes
- Fresh basil
- Baguette slices

Instructions:

1. Slice the baguette and toast until lightly golden.

2. In a bowl, combine chopped cherry tomatoes, sardines, and torn fresh basil leaves.

3. Season with salt, pepper, and a drizzle of olive oil.

4. Spoon the mixture onto the toasted baguette slices.

Sardine and Spinach Stuffed Portobello Mushrooms

Ingredients:

- Sardines (canned)
- Portobello mushrooms
- Spinach
- Garlic cloves
- Parmesan cheese

Instructions:

1. Preheat the oven to 375°F (190°C).
2. Remove the stems from portobello mushrooms and place them on a baking sheet.
3. In a pan, sauté minced garlic until fragrant. Add chopped spinach and cook until wilted.
4. In a bowl, mix the cooked spinach, sardines, and grated Parmesan cheese.
5. Stuff the mushroom caps with the mixture and bake in the preheated oven for 15-20 minutes until the mushrooms are tender and the filling is golden.

Sardine and Potato Croquettes

Ingredients:

- Sardines (canned)
- Potatoes
- Onion
- Breadcrumbs
- Egg

Instructions:

1. Boil the potatoes until tender and mash them in a bowl.

2. Add minced onion, sardines, and egg to the mashed potatoes and mix until combined.

3. Form the mixture into small balls and roll them in breadcrumbs.

4. Fry the croquettes in hot oil until golden brown, about 3 minutes per side.

5. Drain on paper towels before serving.

Sardine and Tomato Pizza

Ingredients:

- Sardines (canned)
- Pizza dough
- Tomato sauce
- Mozzarella cheese
- Fresh basil leaves

Instructions:

1. Preheat the oven to 500°F (260°C).
2. Roll out the pizza dough and spread tomato sauce over it.
3. Top with sardines, mozzarella cheese, and fresh basil leaves.
4. Bake in the preheated oven for 10-15 minutes until the crust is golden and the cheese is bubbly.
5. Serve warm.

Sardine Tacos with Mango Salsa

Ingredients:

- Sardines (canned)
- Soft tacos shells
- Mango
- Red onion
- Cilantro leaves
- Lime juice

Instructions:

1. In a bowl, mix diced mango, finely chopped red onion, and chopped cilantro to make the salsa.

2. Warm the tortillas in a pan or microwave.

3. Place sardines on the tortillas and top with mango salsa.

4. Fold the tortillas and serve as delicious tacos.

Sardine and Rice Stuffed Bell Peppers

Ingredients:

- Sardines (canned)
- Bell peppers
- Cooked rice
- Onion
- Garlic

Instructions:

1. Preheat the oven to 375°F (190°C).
2. Cut off the tops of bell peppers and remove seeds and membranes.
3. In a pan, sauté chopped onion and minced garlic until soft.
4. Mix the sautéed onion and garlic with cooked rice, flaked sardines, salt, and pepper.
5. Stuff the mixture into the bell peppers and place them in a baking dish.
6. Bake for 25-30 minutes until the peppers are tender.

Sardine and Roasted Pepper Sandwich

Ingredients:

- Sardines (canned)
- Roasted red peppers
- Arugula
- Whole wheat bread

Instructions:

1. Toast whole wheat bread slices.
2. Spread sardines on one slice and arrange roasted red peppers and arugula on top.
3. Cover with another slice of bread.
4. Slice the sandwich diagonally and enjoy.

Sardine and Lemon Risotto

Ingredients:

- Sardines (canned)
- Arborio rice
- Lemon
- Vegetable broth
- Parmesan cheese

Instructions:

1. In a saucepan, heat vegetable broth until simmering.

2. In a separate pan, toast Arborio rice for a few minutes.

3. Gradually add the simmering vegetable broth to the rice, stirring continuously until absorbed.

4. Add flaked sardines, zest, juice of a lemon, and grated Parmesan cheese. Stir well.

5. Continue adding broth and stirring until the risotto is creamy and the rice is cooked.

6. Serve immediately, garnished with additional lemon zest if desired.

7-Day Meal Plan

Here is a sample 7-day meal plan to get you started on the sardine diet. Feel free to customize it according to your preferences and dietary needs.

Day 1

Breakfast: Oatmeal with fruit

Lunch: Sardine and Avocado Salad

Dinner: Grilled chicken with steamed vegetables

Day 2

Breakfast: Scrambled eggs with whole-grain toast

Lunch: Sardine and White Bean Dip with vegetable sticks

Dinner: Baked salmon with quinoa

Day 3

Breakfast: Greek yogurt with granola and berries

Lunch: Sardine and Cucumber Salad

Dinner: Grilled steak with sweet potato

Day 4

Breakfast: Smoothie with banana, spinach, and almond milk

Lunch: Sardine and Olive Tapenade on whole-grain bread

Dinner: Roasted turkey with green beans

Day 5

Breakfast: Pancakes with maple syrup

Lunch: Grilled Sardines with Herbs

Dinner: Chicken stir-fry with brown rice

Day 6

Breakfast: French toast with fruit salad

Lunch: Sardine and Tomato Bruschetta

Dinner: Beef stew with whole grain bread

Day 7

Breakfast: Breakfast burrito with eggs, cheese, and salsa

Lunch: Sardine and Spinach Stuffed Portobello Mushrooms

Dinner: Grilled shrimp with pasta

Remember to drink plenty of water and adjust portion sizes based on your dietary needs and goals. Also, feel free to swap out any meals or ingredients to suit your preferences or dietary restrictions. Enjoy!

Conclusion

Congratulations on reaching the end of this comprehensive sardine diet guide! By now, you've gained valuable insights into the numerous benefits and incredible versatility that sardines bring to the table. It's time to take action and embrace this nutritious powerhouse in your daily meals.

Incorporating sardines into your diet offers a multitude of advantages that can transform not only your health but also your overall well-being. From their high protein content promoting satiety and aiding in weight management, to their omega-3 fatty acids supporting heart health and reducing inflammation, sardines are a true superfood.

What sets the sardine diet apart is its adaptability and simplicity. Whether you prefer fresh or canned sardines, these little fish lend themselves to a variety of culinary creations. Get creative in the kitchen and explore the countless possibilities—from salads and wraps to incorporating them into delicious rice bowls or savory fishcakes. Every meal becomes an opportunity to nurture and nourish your body with the goodness of sardines.

Remember, the sardine diet is not just about weight loss or meeting nutritional goals; it's about embracing a sustainable and healthy lifestyle. By making sardines a regular part of your eating routine, you're investing in your long-term health and vitality.

As you embark on this journey, keep in mind a few key tips. First, choose quality sardines that are sustainably sourced and low in sodium. Look for trusted brands or go for fresh options whenever possible. Second, experiment with different recipes and flavors to find what excites your taste buds. Don't be afraid to try new combinations and get adventurous in your culinary pursuits. Lastly, stay consistent and committed to your sardine diet. Incorporate sardines into your weekly meal plans and make it a habit to enjoy their nutritional benefits regularly.

It's important to note that while the sardine diet offers incredible advantages, it's still crucial to maintain a well-rounded and balanced eating plan. Combine sardines with a variety of fruits, vegetables, whole grains, and lean proteins for optimal nutrition.

So, dear reader, are you ready to embark on this exciting journey towards a healthier you? Embrace the sardine diet and witness the positive changes that unfold in your life. From increased energy levels and improved heart health to enhanced weight management and reduced inflammation, the rewards are waiting for you.

It's time to take charge of your nutrition and make the most of what nature has to offer. Let the versatility of sardines open up a world of delectable possibilities that tantalize your taste buds and nourish your body. Remember, you are in control of your health and well-being. By incorporating sardines into your diet, you're choosing a path toward vitality and longevity.

So go ahead, stock up on those cans of sardines, explore new recipes, and savor the flavors of this nutrient-packed fish. Your body will thank you, and you'll be amazed at the transformative power of such a simple addition to your diet.

FAQs

Are sardines a good source of protein?

Yes, sardines are an excellent source of protein. Packed with essential amino acids, they provide approximately 25 grams of high-quality protein per 100 grams. This makes them not only a satisfying addition to any meal but also a nutritious choice for individuals seeking to meet their daily protein requirements. Whether you enjoy them grilled, canned, or in salads, sardines offer a tasty and versatile way to boost your protein intake.

Can sardines help with weight loss?

Sardines are not only low in calories and high in protein, but they also contain essential nutrients such as vitamin D, calcium, and selenium. These nutrients not only support weight loss efforts but also contribute to overall bone health and immune function.

Additionally, the omega-3 fatty acids found in sardines have been linked to improved fat metabolism and have even shown potential benefits for heart health. Incorporating sardines into your diet can be a delicious and nutritious way to enhance your well-being.

Are canned sardines as nutritious as fresh ones?

Canned sardines are not only convenient but also equally nutritionally beneficial as fresh sardines. The canning process effectively preserves its nutritional content, including essential omega-3 fatty acids, vitamins, and minerals, ensuring that you still get all the health benefits.

When selecting canned sardines, opt for lower sodium options and those packed in heart-healthy olive oil to maximize the nutritional advantages and support your overall well-being.

Are sardines safe to eat for pregnant women?

Yes, sardines are not only safe but also highly recommended for pregnant women due to their numerous health benefits. These small, oily fish are packed with omega-3 fatty acids, specifically DHA and EPA, which are essential for the development of the baby's brain and eyes.

Omega-3 fatty acids are known to support optimal cognitive function and visual acuity in infants. Additionally, sardines are also a good source of protein, calcium, and vitamin D, which are important for the overall growth and development of both the mother and the baby. However, it is always advisable to consult with a healthcare professional to get personalized advice based on individual circumstances.

Can sardines help improve heart health?

Sardines are not only delicious but also packed with heart-healthy omega-3 fatty acids. These essential nutrients have been linked to a range of health benefits, including reducing inflammation, lowering cholesterol levels, and improving overall cardiovascular health.

By regularly incorporating sardines into a balanced diet, you can provide your body with the nourishment it needs to support optimal heart function and maintain cardiovascular well-being. So, go ahead and enjoy this flavorful fish as part of your healthy eating routine!

Are there any concerns about mercury levels in sardines?

Sardines, being a low-mercury fish, are a safe choice for regular consumption due to their shorter lifespans and lower mercury accumulation compared to larger predatory fish. This makes them an excellent option for those seeking a healthy seafood choice. However, it is always advisable to maintain a diverse seafood diet to ensure a wide range of nutritional benefits, rather than relying solely on sardines.

Can sardines be included in a gluten-free or dairy-free diet?

Absolutely! Sardines are not only naturally gluten-free and dairy-free, but they are also packed with essential nutrients like omega-3 fatty acids, calcium, and vitamin D. These little fish offer a plethora of health benefits, including supporting heart health, promoting brain function, and strengthening bones.

With their mild flavor and delicate texture, sardines can be effortlessly incorporated into a wide range of recipes, from salads and sandwiches to pasta dishes and spreads. Whether you're looking to boost your omega-3 intake or simply explore new culinary horizons, sardines provide a versatile and nutritious option that caters to those with specific dietary needs.

Resources and Helpful Links

Dighriri, I. M., Alsubaie, A. M., Hakami, F. M., Hamithi, D. M., Alshekh, M. M., Khobrani, F. A., Dalak, F. E., Hakami, A. A., Alsueaadi, E. H., Alsaawi, L. S., Alshammari, S. F., Alqahtani, A. S., Alawi, I. A., Aljuaid, A. A., & Tawhari, M. Q. (2022). Effects of omega-3 polyunsaturated fatty acids on brain functions: a systematic review. Cureus. https://doi.org/10.7759/cureus.30091

Santos, H. O., May, T. L., & Bueno, A. A. (2023). Eating more sardines instead of fish oil supplementation: Beyond omega-3 polyunsaturated fatty acids, a matrix of nutrients with cardiovascular benefits. Frontiers in Nutrition, 10. https://doi.org/10.3389/fnut.2023.1107475

Patel, K. (n.d.). Benefits of omega-3 fatty acids for joint health. www.linkedin.com. https://www.linkedin.com/pulse/benefits-omega-3-fatty-acids-joint-health-dr-kaushik-patel-1f#:~:text=Omega%2D3%20fatty%20acids%20can%20reduce%20the%20risk%20of%20osteoporosis,in%20capsule%20or%20liquid%20form.

Omega-3 and dementia. (n.d.). Alzheimer's Society. https://www.alzheimers.org.uk/about-dementia/risk-factors-and-prevention/omega-3-and-dementia#:~:text=There%20is%20good%20evidence%20that,itself%20is%20behind%20this%20benefit.

Benton, E. (2022). Sardine nutrition facts and health Benefits. Verywell Fit. https://www.verywellfit.com/sardine-nutrition-facts-4428074

Wells, D. (2023, May 30). Are sardines good for you? Healthline. https://www.healthline.com/health/food-nutrition/are-sardines-good-for-you

The Healthy RD. (2023). The 7 Healthiest Sardines Brands in 2023 +Benefits | The Healthy RD. The Healthy RD | Functional Nutrition and Natural Supplements That Support Gut Healing. https://thehealthyrd.com/best-sardines-in-a-can-by-categories-health-benefits/

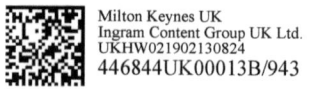

Milton Keynes UK
Ingram Content Group UK Ltd.
UKHW021902130824
446844UK00013B/943